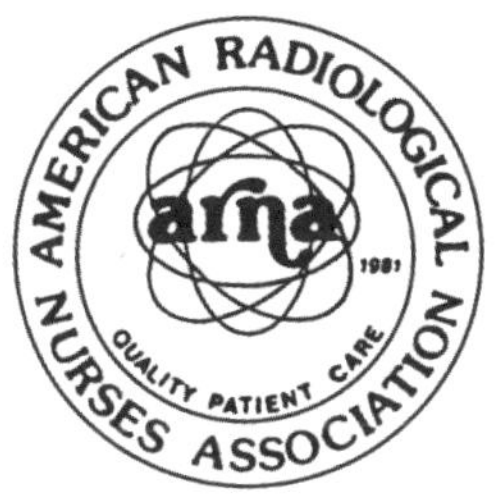

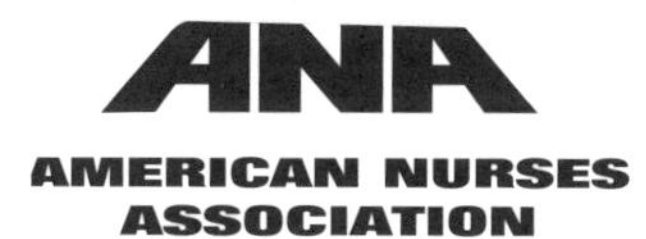

RADIOLOGY NURSING: SCOPE AND STANDARDS OF PRACTICE

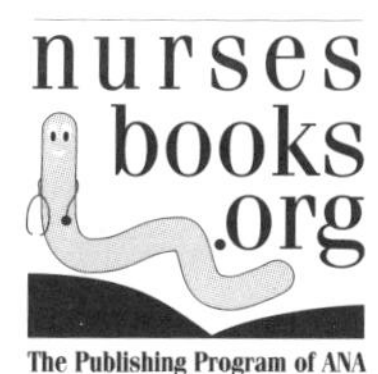

AMERICAN NURSES ASSOCIATION
SILVER SPRING, MARYLAND
2007

Library of Congress Cataloging-in-Publication data

Radiology nursing : scope and standards of practice / American Radiological Nurses Association (ARNA) & American Nurses Association (ANA).
p. ; cm.
Includes bibliographical references and index.
ISBN-13: 978-1-55810-245-3 (pbk.)
ISBN-10: 1-55810-245-0 (pbk.)
1. Nursing—Standards. 2. Radiology, Medical—Standards. I. American Radiological Nurses Association. II. American Nurses Association.
[DNLM: 1. Radiology. 2. Specialties, Nursing. 3. Nursing—standards.
4. Nursing Process—standards. WY 150 R129 2007]

RT85.5.R33 2007
616.07'57—dc22 2006038649

The American Nurses Association (ANA; http://nursingworld.org) is a national professional association. This ANA publication—*Radiology Nursing: Scope and Standards of Practice*—reflects the thinking of the nursing profession on various issues and should be reviewed in conjunction with state board of nursing policies and practices. State law, rules, and regulations govern the practice of nursing, while *Radiology Nursing: Scope and Standards of Practice* guides nurses in the application of their professional skills and responsibilities.

Published by Nursesbooks.org
The Publishing Program of ANA

American Nurses Association
8515 Georgia Avenue, Suite 400
Silver Spring, MD 20910-3492
1-800-274-4ANA
http://www.nursesbooks.org/

ANA is the only full-service professional organization representing the nation's 2.7 million Registered Nurses through its 54 constituent member associations. ANA advances the nursing profession by fostering high standards of nursing practice, promoting the economic and general welfare of nurses in the workplace, projecting a positive and realistic view of nursing, and lobbying the Congress and regulatory agencies on healthcare issues affecting nurses and the public.

The American Radiological Nurses Association (ARNA; http://www.arna.net) is the professional organization representing nurses who practice in diagnostic and therapeutic imaging environments. These nurses provide, promote, and maintain continuity of quality patient care in imaging environments such as general diagnostic, neurointerventional/cardiovascular, interventional, ultrasonography, computerized tomography, nuclear medicine, magnetic resonance, breast health, and radiation oncology.

Design: Scott Bell, Arlington, VA ~ Freedom by Design, Alexandria, VA ~ Stacy Maguire, Sterling, VA ~ *Copyediting*: Lisa Munsat Anthony, Chapel Hill, NC ~ *Indexing & editing*: Steven A. Jent, Denton, TX ~ *Composition*: House of Equations, Inc., Arden, NC ~ *Printing*: McArdle Printing, Upper Marlboro, MD

First printing: November 2006.

ISBN-13: 978-1-55810-236-1 ISBN-10: 1-55810-236-1 SAN: 851-3481
06SSGG 2M 11/06

Acknowledgments

This document was developed by the American Radiological Nurses Association (ARNA) Scope and Standards Revision Task Force. The members of the Task Force gratefully acknowledge the work of others who developed the initial standards of radiological nursing practice published by ARNA in 1998 and those who developed and reviewed drafts of this document.

ARNA Scope and Standards Revision Task Force

Delma Armstrong, BSN, RN, CRN
Teresa Bateman, RN, CRN
Melissa Holbrook, MSN, RN, NP-C
Cindy Sanders, MSN, RN
Leslie Schmidt, MS, RN, CS, NP-C
Paulette Snoby, MPA, BSN, RN, CCRN
Kathy Scheffer, MN, RN, CRN

ARNA Staff

Belinda E. Puetz, PhD, RN
Harriet McClung, BA

ARNA Board of Directors 2003–2004

Kate Little, RN, President
Delma Armstrong, BSN, RN, President-elect
Kathleen Gross, MSN, RN,BC, CRN, Immediate Past President
Sophia Jan, BSN, RN, Treasurer
Kathy Scheffer, BSN, RN, CRN, Secretary
Barbara Sargent, MBA, BSN, RN, Director
Paulette Snoby, MPA, BSN, RN, CCRN, Director
Rhonda Caridi, RN, CRN, Director

ARNA Board of Directors 2004–2005

Delma Armstrong, BSN, RN, CRN, President
Paulette Snoby, MPA, BSN, RN, CCRN, President-elect
Kate Little, RN, Immediate Past President
Sophia Jan, BSN, RN, Treasurer
Kathy Scheffer, MN, RN, CRN, Secretary
Debra Beach, MS, APRN-BC, Director
Rhonda Caridi, RN, CRN, Director
Patrick Glickman, BSN, RN

Contents

Scope of Radiology Nursing Practice

Foundation

Radiology nursing is an exciting and dynamic specialty that combines cutting-edge technology with the art and science of nursing. Visualization of human anatomy and physiology, and a detailed view of the pathophysiology of many disease processes, create a unique practice setting. It is the blending of the nursing commitment to high-quality patient care with compassion for the human condition in this highly technological environment that makes radiology nursing unique.

History of Radiology and Radiology Nursing

Wilhelm Conrad Roentgen, a professor of physics at the University of Würzburg, Germany, discovered X-rays by accident in 1895, hence the name *X*-ray for the unknown. His inadvertent creation of an image on a glass plate while a cathode ray tube was active was a major breakthrough. For the first time, scientists could see structures under the skin. For this discovery, Roentgen won the first Nobel Prize for Physics in 1901. Other early scientists who helped lay the foundation of radiology were Antoine-Henri Becquerel, who discovered the radioactivity of uranium, and Marie and Pierre Curie with their isolation of radium. These three shared the 1903 Nobel Prize for Physics. It would be another 15 years before this knowledge would be used in medicine.

The field of radiology, which exploits short-wavelength electromagnetic radiation that can penetrate matter—the X-ray—has evolved over the years with many technological advancements and an arsenal of imaging modalities. These unique imaging modalities have led to specialties in the radiology field. The use of ultrasound waves, magnetic fields, computer enhancement, and injectable radioactive substances has created other means to diagnose and treat disease processes and further advance the ability to understand the human condition.

Radiation has been studied extensively, and research on its effects, its usefulness, and its dangers continues. This technological progress has placed new demands on healthcare workers and increased the need for highly trained radiologists, nurses, and technologists working as a team to ensure patient safety.

Acknowledgment of the uniqueness of the practice setting and the specialized body of knowledge required to care for patients in this arena led to the foundation of the American Radiological Nurses Association (ARNA). In 1980, the call went out in *RN Magazine* for radiology nurses to organize. The following year 35 radiology nurses from 15 states met in conjunction with the 67th Scientific Assembly and Annual Meeting of the Radiological Society of North America (RSNA). In November, to advance their practice and institute standards of care, they established the American Radiological Nurses Association.

Partnering with RSNA was a strategic move for ARNA; it allowed the nurses to share speakers and facilities with the medical community for their educational venues. ARNA also sought recognition from other nursing organizations and soon joined the Nursing Organization Liaison Forum/National Federation of Specialty Nursing Organization (NOLF/NFSNO). This allowed ARNA to have a voice in specialty nursing issues. ARNA was also recognized by the American Nurses Association (ANA) as a specialty nursing association. In reaction to the nursing shortage of the 1990s, NOLF/NFSNO dissolved and reformed as the Nursing Organizations Alliance. ARNA has been represented at each meeting of this new organization.

Another influence on the growth and development of radiological nursing was the Joint Commission on Accreditation of Healthcare Organizations (JCAHO). JCAHO mandates prompted the organization of radiology departments, to the advantage of radiology nurses. JCAHO wanted to see patients receive the same level of care in diagnostic and procedure areas that they would receive in the inpatient unit. Procedural sedation also became a major patient safety focus in the late 1990s. JCAHO also wanted to see nurses directly supervised by nurses. This led to more radiology nurses and more supervision by nurses with radiology experience. Many hospitals had to manage this requirement creatively by cross-training perianesthesia care units (PACUs) and transport nurses to cover radiology areas when required.

More external changes in reimbursement through Diagnostic Related Groupings (DRGs) and Medicare, with private insurance following closely, meant that procedures formerly considered surgical and requiring hospitalization were re-conceived as minimally invasive procedures that could be performed on outpatients in the radiology department. Smaller incisions, less pain, and shorter recovery times led radiology in a new direction. Inferior vena cava (IVC) filters, internal ureteral stenting, percutaneous drainage tubes, central venous access for dialysis, and oncologic treatments were a few of the innovative procedures that emerged.

Technological advances and organizational changes expanded the role of the radiology nurse to meet the demands of patient care and safety in the radiology department. Just as surgical patients receive nursing intervention early in their hospital stays, patients undergoing care in the radiology department require the radiology nurse's attention and care from the time a test or procedure is requested until the patient is discharged.

These changes in the practice setting, and growing awareness of the unique and specialized knowledge needed to perform competently there, led ARNA to produce its first certification exam in 1998. *Core Curriculum for Radiological Nursing* (Morgan & Nunnelee, 1999) soon followed to serve as a guide for nurses coming into this new field of practice.

With the new millennium came increased emphasis on organizational development and change. ARNA recruited a management company experienced in nursing organizations of various sizes. Many changes were made to streamline the work of the organization and to best use ARNA's resources. In 2002 ARNA was accredited as a Provider Unit by the ANCC Commission on Accreditation.

This commitment to the core ideology that led to the formation of ARNA continues to this day and is reflected in the mission of ARNA: *To foster the growth of radiology nurses who advance the standard of care.*

ARNA's core values—the essential and enduring principles that guide an organization—are found in its strategic plan formulated in 2004:

- Commitment to professionalism
- Responsiveness to technological advances
- Commitment to being the leaders in a constantly evolving environment

The ARNA strategic plan also includes a long-term goal for the association: to be *the* source for standards of nursing care in *any* imaging environment. These standards of radiology nursing practice have been formulated to achieve that goal.

Populations Served

Radiology patients range in age from newborn to geriatric; they may present with actual or potential alterations in health status in one or more body systems. The radiology nurse knows that patients may also experience accompanying mental, emotional, or spiritual distress. Radiology nurses are skilled in the initial treatment of alterations that may result from radiology procedures. These alterations may include contrast-induced allergies, changes in hemodynamic status, complications from procedural sedation, or a variety of other side effects. Radiology nurses diagnose and treat the range of human responses within their practice settings, scope of licensure, and available resources. Radiology nurses prioritize patient care activities based on patient acuity, risk factors, safety needs, the urgent or expedient nature of the procedure, and available resources. Radiology nurses serve their community as parish nurses, by teaching breast self exams, by advocating for early screening mammograms for high risk patients, and as partners in the Society of Interventional Radiologists "Legs for Life" peripheral vascular screening program.

Practice Settings

The practice setting offers unique challenges to radiology nursing. Radiology nursing practice takes place in settings which range across the continuum of care: inpatient and outpatient facilities in hospitals varying in size from small community facilities to university medical centers; same-day or limited-stay facilities; freestanding outpatient centers; and ambulatory radiology clinics.

Radiology is a high-volume specialty in which rapid throughput is desirable. Because of this rapid pace, radiology nurse–patient interactions may be single or multiple brief encounters. Radiology nurses work in practice settings in which there are often simultaneous demands competing for their services. This requires the radiology nurse to partner with other clinical nurses to ensure patient safety and appropriate care. This may include the use of the Perianesthesia Care Unit (PACU) for recovery from procedural sedation or the Intensive Care Unit (ICU) for close follow-up monitoring after renal artery angioplasty or arterial thrombolysis.

The radiology nurse's activities vary depending on the practice setting and the nursing staff available. In smaller facilities one nurse may cover all the patient care needs of the department, while larger facilities may employ an entire department of nurses. Patient advocacy and education are prime responsibilities of the nurse, whether a staff of one or many. Coordination of care with other healthcare team members is essential for a successful patient encounter. This encounter often begins with a phone call from the radiology nurse to the patient at home before a scheduled procedure. This call enables the nurse to screen the patient clinically, ensure that the patient and family understand the procedure, and answer their questions.

Definition and Description of Radiology Nursing

Radiology nursing is the assessment, care planning, and direct care of patients before, during, and after diagnostic and therapeutic imaging procedures. Radiology nurses always advocate for patients; they are frequently the voice of those unable to speak for themselves. Safety of the patient, as well as of the staff, is a primary concern.

Protocols and patient guidelines are based on best evidence-based practice. Such research is ongoing and performed in conjunction with other radiological organizations such as the American College of Radiology (ACR) and the American Society of Radiology Technologists (ASRT). Research is continuing to seek the best method to decrease the nephrotoxicity of contrast agents in high-risk patients. For example, studies have shown that contrast allergies are not positively linked to shellfish allergies as previously believed. Prescreening patients at risk is a major role of the radiology nurse, and staying current in the most recent research will ensure patient safety.

Radiology nurses influence patient care in a variety of settings, and the nursing roles in radiology may be as diverse as the specialty itself. Nurses may be employed as administrators, nursing recruiters, educators, performance improvement or risk management specialists, and marketers. Subspecialty areas include diagnostic imaging, vascular and interventional procedures (sometimes called *special procedures*), computed tomography scanning, nuclear medicine including positron emission tomographic (PET) scanning, ultrasound, magnetic resonance imaging, breast imaging, radiation oncology, lithotripsy, cardiac catheterization, and related research, education, marketing, and consulting areas.

Radiology nurses work with and teach student nurses, residents, and medical students as they rotate through radiology. Many institutions include radiology nursing as a permanent part of new nurse orientation and have created nursing guides to radiology procedures to aid staff nurses in planning patient care.

Advanced practice nurses have a place in radiology practice whether assisting in clinic evaluations, conducting research, or performing follow-up care for patients who have undergone complex invasive procedures.

In accordance with *Nursing's Social Policy Statement* (ANA, 2003), radiology nurses address issues of health and wellness with patients during therapeutic and interventional procedures in the radiology department. They work within institutional and other constraints to ensure that the nursing care they provide is of the highest quality and is targeted toward the needs of individual patients.

Radiology nursing continues to advance as a specialty area of practice with a distinct body of knowledge that is increasingly evidence-based. It bases its ethics on *Code of Ethics for Nurses with Interpretive Statements* (ANA, 2001). The radiology nurse adhering to this professional code acknowledges the patient's right to privacy and confidentiality, to be informed, and to be treated with dignity. Furthermore, the radiology nurse recognizes the patient as a unique individual who is part of a structure that involves family, community, and society.

Both the registered radiology nurse and the advanced practice radiology registered nurse respect the patient's cultural beliefs, acknowledge the patient's diversity, and honor the patient's individuality. In this way, these nurses ensure that the care they provide is non-judgmental and non-discriminatory, regardless of the patient's characteristics or attributes, such as religion or lifestyle.

The radiology nurse serves as a patient advocate and helps the patient to make decisions regarding health care. In the radiology environment, radiology nurses promote professional ethics on their part and on the part of those with whom they work (e.g., radiologists, radiology technicians, other radiology nurses). Radiology nurses also promote their own professional integrity and that of others.

The scope of radiology nursing practice is guided by federal and state laws and regulations, clinical research, the code of ethics (ANA, 2001), best practices that are evidence-based, professional organizations, standards of practice (ANA, 2004), and position statements and guidelines developed by ARNA and other specialty organizations, such as the Association of periOperative Registered Nurses (AORN).

Radiology nurses require specialized knowledge and clinical skills to deal with the possible effects of radiological interventions on patients from infants to the elderly. In addition to standard nursing education and clinical experience, a greater understanding of the following subjects facilitates radiology nursing practice:

- Adaptation and change process
- Coping mechanisms
- Cultural and spiritual diversity
- Growth and development, to include both pediatric and elder care
- Human sexuality
- Communication skills
- Therapeutic use of self
- Patient advocacy
- Safety
- Infection control principles and practices
- Informed consent
- Radiation safety principles and practices
- Stages of pregnancy and fetal development, and risks of radiation exposure
- Radiological emergencies and appropriate initial interventions
- Procedural sedation: risks, benefits, complications, and reversal agents
- Pain control and symptom management
- Positioning for optimum comfort, radiation protection, and procedural needs

- Risks and complications associated with contrast media administration
- Preparation for individual procedures, educating and screening for these procedures
- Risks and complications associated with procedures
- Technological advances that affect patient care and departmental operations

Radiology nurses use the *nursing process* in planning for and providing care to patients undergoing diagnostic and therapeutic imaging procedures. The nursing process includes assessment, diagnosis, identifying outcomes, creating a plan of care, implementing the plan of care, and evaluating the effectiveness of interventions based on patient responses. The plan of care addresses age-appropriate, developmentally appropriate, culturally appropriate, family-centered, and environmentally sensitive issues. Radiology nursing roles include, but are not limited to, patient advocate, care coordinator, caregiver, role model, educator, resource person, consultant, communication liaison, manager, administrator, and researcher. Radiology nurses serve as part of an interdisciplinary team that includes radiologists, radiological technologists, primary care physicians, inpatient and home health nurses, the patient and family members, and others. Radiology nurses focus on the patient and the patient's responses to radiological interventions or physiologic changes while in the radiology department or under the care of the radiologist or radiology nurse.

Radiology Nurse Practice Levels

Radiology nursing is diverse and dynamic. Radiology nurses assume roles based on basic nursing preparation and scope of practice as determined by licensure, specialized informal and formal education, clinical experience, interest, talent, personal experience, and the nature of the patient population. Radiology nurses may be generalists or advanced practice nurses who work in various healthcare settings. At the current time, registered nurses with a Diploma, Associate degree, Baccalaureate, or Master of Science in Nursing practice in radiology settings. Licensed practical or vocational nurses also practice in some radiology settings within the more limited scope of their licensure.

Radiology Nurse Generalist

The radiology nurse generalist is a licensed registered nurse who demonstrates clinical skills and knowledge in radiology nursing and imaging technologies. The radiology nurse generalist should possess the basic knowledge and skills to complete activities such as the following:

- Apply appropriate theory and evidence-based practice as the basis for decision-making in radiology nursing practice.
- Use nursing and radiology procedural knowledge to anticipate and plan for patient care needs in the radiology environment. The radiology nurse is expert in assessing and treating anxiety, pain, claustrophobia, and underlying disease conditions (they care for GI bleeders, patients with pulmonary emboli, seizure disorders, cardiac disease, acute gallbladder or hepatic conditions, and renal obstruction).
- Provide expert care related to tubes and devices located in the radiology department. The radiology nurse knows the potential risks and complications from radiology procedures and can assist in the initial treatment of adverse effects particularly associated with contrast media administration and in the treatment of these complications.
- Understand the pharmacology of medications and recognize special considerations related to drugs and pharmacologic agents rarely used in other areas—for example, cholecysteine, arterial nitroglycerine infusions for venous spasm, intravenous glucagons to reduce peristalsis during gastric procedures, procedural sedation which evolves into mild and moderate sedation, pain and anxiolytic medications for immediate and long-term relief, adenosine and dobutamine for cardiac pharmacologic stress testing, and diuretics and other cardiac beta blockers used to facilitate diagnostic testing.
- Understand and apply radiation safety principles and serve as a resource to other healthcare personnel on radiology patient care.
- Facilitate a multidisciplinary approach that enhances continuity of care and patient care outcomes by collaborating with other healthcare providers. This includes delegating appropriate aspects of patient care to qualified personnel. The radiology nurse has expanded the radiology team:

Radiologist + Radiology Technologist (RT) = Partnership

Radiologist + RT+ RN = *Team*

This requires a reorientation of the radiology department, primarily facilitated by the addition of nursing to the team. The radiology nurse is an essential specialist and resource who enhances both patient and department outcomes.

- Assist in identification of pertinent issues such as patient care, safety, and infection control and provide informal and formal education on these issues to radiology staff. The radiology nurse is essential to developing and implementing ongoing performance improvement processes.
- Participate in evaluation processes to enhance professional performance, including peer review. The radiology nurse must assume personal responsibility for continuing education and professional growth.
- Understand the research process, be able to participate in data collection, and incorporate pertinent findings into practice. As interventional and research efforts increase, nurses move into positions of responsibility supporting these efforts, recruiting and following subjects, and coordinating studies.

The nursing process is a systematic, deliberate problem-solving approach to meeting the health care and nursing needs of patients)—assessment, diagnosis, planning, implementation, evaluation, outcomes identification—has expanded the ability of the radiology department to assess the impact of changes in policy and personnel, and has helped put the patient first in the priorities of the department. The use of the nursing process for patients undergoing diagnostic and therapeutic imaging procedures includes:

- Collection of ongoing data
- Synthesis and analysis of data to determine outcomes
- Development of an age-appropriate plan of care
- Implementation of the nursing plan
- Evaluation of the patient's responses to the plan
- Reassessment and revision of the plan and goals as indicated

Radiology nurses are the primary patient advocates in the radiology department; they often speak for patients who cannot speak for themselves, they protect the patients' privacy and dignity, and they ensure focus on the patient. That is, they provide nursing *care*. They also are attuned to the language, ethnic, religious, and sexual diversity of patients.

Such a role helps maintain patient confidentiality while communicating pertinent clinical data. The nurse must also provide health education and procedural teaching to patients and significant others before, during, and after procedures. Radiology nurses must possess excellent communication skills. Positive personal interactions and flexibility are key to providing clear instruction and communication with patients and family members as well as other members of the radiology team.

Radiology Advanced Practice Registered Nurse

The radiology advanced practice registered nurse has a master's or doctoral degree and has been recognized and credentialed as an advanced practice registered nurse in the state in which they practice.

The increasing severity and complexity of patient illnesses in acute care settings drive the development of advanced radiology nursing roles as the specialty continues to evolve and more radiology nurses attain graduate degrees. The radiology advanced practice registered nurse may function in a variety of roles and settings that include, but are not limited to, the following: clinician, supervisor, administrator, educator, consultant, researcher, performance improvement specialist, risk manager, care coordinator, or communication liaison.

In the direct patient care setting, these nurses may work as clinical nurse specialists or nurse practitioners. They base their decisions on nursing theory combined with research and clinical knowledge. Radiology advanced practice nurses in clinical roles demonstrate a high level of autonomy, rendering complex clinical decisions and initiating treatment regimens including treatment for contrast-related events, peripheral vascular disease management, and follow-up care after therapeutic interventions. They conduct comprehensive peri-procedural health assessments and demonstrate expert skill in diagnosis and treatment of complex responses of individuals, families, and communities to actual or potential health problems. They function in collegial relationships with nursing peers and physicians. The radiology advanced practice nurse acts as a resource for other nurses, physicians, and radiology technologists.

All radiology advanced practice nurses work within the larger health-care environment. They need to be current and competent in direct patient care and comfortable serving as change agents and leaders in their practice setting.

Certification

Certification is a process whereby a certifying organization or governing agency validates a registered nurse's qualifications, knowledge, and scope of practice in a defined clinical or functional area of nursing. A nurse achieves certification by meeting eligibility requirements determined by the governing agency and by passing a written examination on current practice standards in the specialized practice setting. Through this process, the certifying agency acknowledges to the nurse, the nurse's colleagues, and the general public that the individual has mastered the body of knowledge that pertains to the nursing specialty.

The Radiologic Nursing Certification Board (RNCB) has established eligibility requirements, created an examination for initial certification, and identified a re-certification process for recognition as a Certified Radiological Nurse (CRN). Upon passing the examination, the nurse may use the initials CRN in addition to licensing and educational designations. The CRN designation attests that the nurse has demonstrated in-depth knowledge of the field of radiology nursing. Specific information about this specialty certification is available from ARNA at http://www.arna.net. An advanced level certification for radiology nursing is not available at this time.

Nurse practitioners and clinical nurse specialists may be required to have professional certification in order to practice. This certification denotes their advanced practice status and is administered by governing bodies other than the RNCB, such as the American Nurses Credentialing Center (ANCC).

Issues and Opportunities

One of the most pressing issues facing ARNA is the lack of dedicated radiology nurses in all imaging suites across the country. It is ARNA's belief that where patient care is rendered, nursing must be present. Radiology departments have become highly specialized and technologically advanced. Similarly, the complexity and acuity level of patient conditions have risen. Radiology nurses skilled in critical care and possessing specialized knowledge in the field are imperative to ensure safe and effective outcomes for our patients.

ARNA has developed orientation materials that cover the appropriate content needed to prepare nurses for radiology specialty practice. There are no formal academic programs yet. The second edition of *Core Curriculum for Radiological Nursing* is a critical information resource until such programs can be developed and implemented.

Summary

Quality care for all patients is a primary responsibility of nurses. The standards of care and standards of professional practice can help the nurse set goals for professional growth in the specialty of radiology nursing practice.

The art of nursing also has an essence that is not defined or measured by scientific analysis; standards of caring, compassion, commitment, and nursing intuition must be established by each radiology nurse to promote the highest level of patient care.

STANDARDS OF RADIOLOGY NURSING PRACTICE STANDARDS OF PRACTICE

STANDARD 1. ASSESSMENT

The radiology registered nurse collects comprehensive data pertinent to the patient's health and situation.

Measurement Criteria:

The radiology registered nurse:

- Collects data in a systematic and ongoing process. For example, health history pertinent to the radiology environment, which can include, but is not limited to:
  - *Medical history*:
    - Ability to lie flat without discomfort
    - Ability to follow verbal instructions
    - Allergies and type of allergic reaction
    - Renal function if the patient is over age 65 and is to receive IV contrast
    - Adverse reactions to procedural sedation
    - Past experiences with pain medications and pain management
  - *Surgical history*:
    - Pacemaker, cochlear implant, metal implants, implantable electronic devices of any sort
    - Recent surgeries
  - *Psychosocial history*:
    - Significant other identified
    - Cultural considerations identified and addressed
    - Any past claustrophobia
    - Substance abuse history
    - Needle phobia (belonephobia)

Continued ►

    - Past experiences that influence ability to relax or cooperate
    - Accidents or injuries
        - Metal fragments in the eye or face (MRI)
    - Communicable disease
        - May require special environmental adjustments and scheduling
    - Safety
        - Risk of falls
- Prioritizes data collection activities based on the patient's immediate condition, or the anticipated needs of the patient or situation.
- Involves the patient, family, other healthcare providers, and environment, as appropriate, in holistic data collection.
- Uses appropriate evidence-based assessment techniques and instruments in collecting pertinent data.
- Uses analytical models and problem-solving tools.
- Synthesizes available data, information, and knowledge relevant to the situation to identify patterns and variances.
- Documents relevant data in a retrievable format.
- Uses developmentally and age-appropriate assessment techniques when the patient is a child or an elder.
- Uses age- and size-appropriate instruments to collect assessment data when the patient is a child or an elder.

Additional Measurement Criteria for the Advanced Practice Radiology Registered Nurse:

The advanced practice radiology registered nurse:

- Initiates and interprets diagnostic tests and procedures relevant to the patient's current status.
- Bases assessment techniques on current research.

STANDARD 2. DIAGNOSIS

The radiology registered nurse analyzes the assessment data to determine the diagnoses or issues.

Measurement Criteria:

The radiology registered nurse:

- Derives the diagnoses or issues based on assessment data.
- Validates the diagnoses or issues with the patient, family, and other healthcare providers when possible and appropriate.
- Makes diagnoses that are developmentally and age-appropriate. These include growth and development and family dynamics as applicable when the patient is a child or an elder.
- Documents diagnoses or issues in a manner that facilitates the determination of the expected outcomes and plan.

Additional Measurement Criteria for the Advanced Practice Radiology Registered Nurse:

The advanced practice radiology registered nurse:

- Systematically compares clinical findings with normal and abnormal variations and developmental events in formulating a differential diagnosis.
- Uses complex data and information obtained during interview, examination, and diagnostic procedures in identifying diagnoses.
- Assists staff in developing and maintaining competency in the diagnostic process.

STANDARD 3. OUTCOMES IDENTIFICATION

The radiology registered nurse identifies expected outcomes for a plan individualized to the patient and situation.

Measurement Criteria:

The radiology registered nurse:

- Involves the patient, family, and other healthcare providers in formulating expected outcomes when possible and appropriate.
- Derives culturally appropriate expected outcomes from the diagnoses.
- Considers associated risks, benefits, costs, current scientific evidence, and clinical expertise when formulating expected and realistic outcomes.
- Defines expected outcomes in terms of the patient, patient values, ethical considerations, environment, or situation with such considerations as associated risks, benefits and costs, and current scientific evidence.
- Includes a time estimate for attainment of expected outcomes.
- Develops expected outcomes that provide direction for continuity of care.
- Ensures that outcomes are developmentally and age-appropriate when the patient is a child or an elder.
- Modifies expected outcomes based on changes in the status of the patient or evaluation of the situation.
- Documents expected outcomes as measurable goals.

Additional Measurement Criteria for the Advanced Practice Radiology Registered Nurse:

The advanced practice radiology registered nurse:

- Identifies expected outcomes that incorporate scientific evidence and are achievable through implementation of evidence-based practices.

- Identifies expected outcomes that incorporate cost and clinical effectiveness, patient satisfaction, and continuity and consistency among providers.
- Supports the use of clinical guidelines linked to positive patient outcomes.

STANDARD 4. PLANNING

The radiology registered nurse develops a plan that prescribes strategies and alternatives to attain expected outcomes.

Measurement Criteria:

The radiology registered nurse:

- Develops an individualized plan considering patient characteristics and the situation.
- Develops the plan in conjunction with the patient, family, and others, as appropriate.
- Includes strategies in the plan that address each of the identified diagnoses or issues, which may include strategies for promotion and restoration of health and prevention of illness, injury, and disease.
- Provides for continuity in the plan.
- Incorporates an implementation pathway or timeline in the plan.
- Establishes the plan priorities with the patient, family, and others as appropriate.
- Uses the plan to provide direction to other members of the healthcare team.
- Defines the plan to reflect current statutes, rules and regulations, and standards.
- Integrates current trends and research affecting care in the planning process.
- Considers the economic impact of the plan.
- Uses standardized language or recognized terminology to document the plan.

Additional Measurement Criteria for the Advanced Practice Radiology Registered Nurse:

The advanced practice radiology registered nurse:

- Identifies assessment, diagnostic strategies, and therapeutic interventions in the plan that reflect current evidence, including data, research, literature, and expert clinical knowledge.

- Selects or designs strategies to meet the multifaceted needs of complex patients.
- Includes the synthesis of patients' values and beliefs regarding nursing and medical therapies in the plan.
- Participates in the design and development of multidisciplinary and interdisciplinary processes to address the situation or issue.
- Contributes to the development and continuous improvement of organizational systems that support the planning process.
- Supports the integration of clinical, human, and financial resources to enhance and complete the decision-making process.

STANDARD 5. IMPLEMENTATION
The radiology registered nurse implements the strategies in the identified plan.

Measurement Criteria:

The radiology registered nurse:

- Implements the plan in a safe and timely manner.
- Documents implementation and any modifications, including changes to or omissions from the identified plan.
- Uses evidence-based interventions and treatments specific to the diagnosis or problem.
- Ensures that the interventions are developmentally and age-appropriate and family-centered when the patient is a child or an elder.
- Uses community resources and systems to implement the plan.
- Collaborates with nursing colleagues and others to implement the plan.

Additional Measurement Criteria for the Advanced Practice Radiology Registered Nurse:

The advanced practice radiology registered nurse:

- Facilitates the use of systems and community resources to implement the plan.
- Supports collaboration with nursing colleagues and other disciplines to implement the plan.
- Incorporates new knowledge and strategies to initiate change in nursing care practices if desired outcomes are not achieved.

STANDARD 5A. COORDINATION OF CARE

The radiology registered nurse coordinates care delivery in a variety of radiological settings.

Measurement Criteria:

The radiology registered nurse:

- Acts as a case manager to ensure that the patient with multiple radiological studies or interventions receives these in the most efficient manner.
- Negotiates specialized care needs with the patient, family, appropriate systems, outside agencies, and providers prior to radiological intervention.
- Coordinates implementation of the plan.
- Documents the coordination of care.

Measurement Criteria for the Advanced Practice Radiology registered nurse:

The advanced practice radiology registered nurse:

- Provides leadership in the coordination of multidisciplinary health care for integrated delivery of patient care services.
- Synthesizes data and information to prescribe necessary system and community support measures, including environmental modifications.
- Coordinates system and community resources that enhance delivery of care across continuums.

STANDARD 5B. HEALTH TEACHING AND HEALTH PROMOTION

The radiology registered nurse employs strategies to promote health and a safe environment.

Measurement Criteria:

The radiology registered nurse:

- Provides health teaching that addresses such topics as healthy lifestyles, risk-reducing behaviors, developmental needs, activities of daily living, and preventive self-care.
- Provides health teaching that ensures a safe environment through modality-specific pre-screening and recognition of inherent risks associated with diagnostic and therapeutic imaging and procedures.
- Uses health promotion and health teaching methods appropriate to the situation and the patient's developmental level, learning needs, readiness, ability to learn, language preference, and culture whether a child or an elder.
- Seeks opportunities for feedback and evaluation of the effectiveness of the strategies used.

Additional Measurement Criteria for the Advanced Practice Radiology Registered Nurse:

The advanced practice radiology registered nurse:

- Synthesizes empirical evidence on risk behaviors, learning theories, behavioral change theories, motivational theories, epidemiology, and other related theories and frameworks when designing health information and patient education.
- Designs health information and patient education based on current scientific knowledge and research and appropriate to the patient's developmental level, learning needs, readiness to learn, and cultural values and beliefs.
- Evaluates health information resources, such as the Internet, in the area of practice for accuracy, readability, and comprehensibility to help patients access quality health information.

STANDARD 5C. CONSULTATION

The advanced practice radiology registered nurse provides consultation to influence the identified plan, enhance the abilities of others, and effect change.

Additional Measurement Criteria for the Advanced Practice Radiology Registered Nurse:

The advanced practice radiology registered nurse:

- Synthesizes clinical data, theoretical frameworks, and evidence when providing consultation.
- Facilitates the effectiveness of a consultation by involving the patient in decision-making, negotiating role responsibilities, and ensuring that understanding is reached.
- Communicates consultation recommendations that facilitate change.

STANDARD 5D. PRESCRIPTIVE AUTHORITY AND TREATMENT

The advanced practice radiology registered nurse uses prescriptive authority, procedures, referrals, treatments, and therapies in accordance with state and federal laws and regulations.

Measurement Criteria for the Advanced Practice Radiology Registered Nurse:

The advanced practice radiology registered nurse:

- Prescribes evidence-based treatments, therapies, and procedures considering the patient's comprehensive healthcare needs.
- Prescribes pharmacological agents based on a current knowledge of pharmacology and physiology.
- Prescribes specific pharmacological agents and treatments based on clinical indicators, the patient's status and needs, and the results of diagnostic and laboratory tests.
- Evaluates therapeutic and potential adverse effects of pharmacological and non-pharmacological treatments.
- Provides patients with information about intended effects and potential adverse effects of proposed prescriptive therapies.
- Provides information about costs and alternative treatments and procedures, as appropriate.

STANDARD 6. EVALUATION

The radiology registered nurse evaluates progress toward attainment of outcomes.

Measurement Criteria:

The radiology registered nurse:

- Conducts a systematic, ongoing, and criterion-based evaluation of the outcomes in relation to the structures and processes prescribed by the plan and the indicated timeline.
- Includes the patient and others involved in the care or situation in the evaluative process.
- Evaluates the effectiveness of the planned strategies in relation to patient responses and the attainment of the expected outcomes.
- Documents the results of the evaluation.
- Uses ongoing assessment data to revise the diagnoses, outcomes, the plan, and the implementation as needed.
- Disseminates the results to the patient and others involved in the care or situation, as appropriate, in accordance with state and federal laws and regulations.

Additional Measurement Criteria for the Advanced Practice Radiology Registered Nurse:

The advanced practice radiology registered nurse:

- Evaluates the accuracy of the diagnosis and effectiveness of the interventions in relationship to the patient's attainment of expected outcomes.
- Synthesizes the results of the evaluation analyses to determine the impact of the plan on the affected patients, families, groups, communities, and institutions.
- Uses the results of the evaluation analyses to make or recommend process or structural changes including policy, procedure or protocol documentation, as appropriate.

STANDARDS OF PROFESSIONAL PERFORMANCE

STANDARD 7. QUALITY OF PRACTICE
The radiology registered nurse systematically enhances the quality and effectiveness of nursing practice.

Measurement Criteria:

The radiology registered nurse:

- Demonstrates quality by documenting the application of the nursing process in a responsible, accountable, and ethical manner.
- Uses the results of quality improvement activities to initiate changes in nursing practice and in the healthcare delivery system.
- Uses creativity and innovation in nursing practice to improve care delivery.
- Incorporates new knowledge to initiate changes in nursing practice if desired outcomes are not achieved.
- Participates in quality improvement activities. Such activities may include:
  - Identifying aspects of practice important for quality monitoring.
  - Using indicators developed to monitor quality and effectiveness of nursing practice.
  - Collecting data to monitor quality and effectiveness of nursing practice.
  - Analyzing quality data to identify opportunities for improving nursing practice.
  - Formulating recommendations to improve nursing practice or outcomes.
  - Implementing activities to enhance the quality of nursing practice.
  - Developing, implementing, and evaluating policies, procedures, and guidelines to improve the quality of practice.

Continued ▶

- Participating on interdisciplinary teams to evaluate clinical care or health services.
- Participating in efforts to minimize costs and unnecessary duplication.
- Analyzing factors related to safety, satisfaction, effectiveness, and cost–benefit options.
- Analyzing organizational systems for barriers.
- Implementing processes to remove or decrease barriers in organizational systems.

Additional Measurement Criteria for the Advanced Practice Radiology Registered Nurse:

The advanced practice radiology registered nurse:

- Obtains and maintains professional certification.
- Designs quality improvement initiatives.
- Implements initiatives to evaluate the need for change.
- Evaluates the practice environment and quality of nursing care delivered in relation to existing evidence, identifying opportunities for the generation and use of research.

STANDARD 8. EDUCATION

The radiology registered nurse attains knowledge and competency that reflects current nursing practice.

Measurement Criteria:

The radiology registered nurse:

- Participates in ongoing educational activities related to appropriate knowledge bases and professional issues.
- Demonstrates a commitment to lifelong learning through self-reflection and inquiry to identify learning needs.
- Seeks experiences that reflect current practice in order to maintain skills and competence in clinical practice or role performance.
- Acquires knowledge and skills appropriate to the specialty area, practice setting, role, or situation.
- Maintains professional records that provide evidence of competency and lifelong learning.
- Seeks experiences and formal and independent learning activities to maintain and develop clinical and professional skills and knowledge.

Additional Measurement Criteria for the Advanced Practice Radiology Registered Nurse:

The advanced practice radiology registered nurse:

- Uses current healthcare research findings and other evidence to expand clinical knowledge, enhance role performance, and increase knowledge of professional issues.

STANDARD 9. PROFESSIONAL PRACTICE EVALUATION

The radiology registered nurse evaluates one's own nursing practice in relation to professional practice standards and guidelines, relevant statutes, rules, and regulations.

Measurement Criteria:

The radiology registered nurse's practice reflects the application of knowledge of current practice standards, guidelines, statutes, rules, and regulations. The radiology registered nurse:

- Provides age-appropriate care in a culturally and ethnically sensitive manner.
- Engages in self-evaluation of practice on a regular basis, identifying areas of strength as well as areas in which professional development would be beneficial.
- Obtains informal feedback regarding one's own practice from patients, peers, professional colleagues, and others.
- Participates in systematic peer review as appropriate.
- Takes action to achieve goals identified during the evaluation process.
- Provides rationale for practice beliefs, decisions, and actions as part of the informal and formal evaluation processes.

Additional Measurement Criteria for the Advanced Practice Radiology Registered Nurse:

The advanced practice radiology registered nurse:

- Engages in a formal process seeking feedback regarding one's own practice from patients, peers, professional colleagues, and others.

STANDARD 10. COLLEGIALITY

The radiology registered nurse interacts with and contributes to the professional development of peers and colleagues.

Measurement Criteria:

The radiology registered nurse:

- Shares knowledge and skills with peers and colleagues as evidenced by such activities as patient care conferences or presentations at formal or informal meetings.
- Provides peers with feedback regarding their practice and role performance.
- Interacts with peers and colleagues to enhance one's own professional nursing practice and role performance.
- Maintains compassionate and caring relationships with peers and colleagues.
- Contributes to an environment that is conducive to the education of healthcare professionals.
- Contributes to a supportive and healthy work environment.

Additional Measurement Criteria for the Advanced Practice Radiology Registered Nurse:

The advanced practice radiology registered nurse:

- Models expert practice to interdisciplinary team members and healthcare consumers.
- Mentors other radiology registered nurses and colleagues as appropriate.
- Participates with interdisciplinary teams that contribute to role development and advanced nursing practice and health care.
- Participates in professional activities.
- Contributes to an environment that is conducive to clinical education of other healthcare providers and acts as teacher, mentor, and preceptor, as appropriate.

STANDARD 11. COLLABORATION
The radiology registered nurse collaborates with patient, family, and others in the conduct of nursing practice.

Measurement Criteria:

The radiology registered nurse:

- Communicates with patient, family, and healthcare providers regarding patient care and the nurse's role in the provision of that care.
- Collaborates in creating a documented plan focused on outcomes and decisions related to care and delivery of services that indicates communication with patients, families, and others.
- Partners with others to effect change and generate positive outcomes through knowledge of the patient or situation.
- Documents referrals, including provisions for continuity of care.

Additional Measurement Criteria for the Advanced Practice Radiology Registered Nurse:

The advanced practice radiology registered nurse:

- Partners with other disciplines to enhance patient care through interdisciplinary activities such as education, consultation, management, technological development, or research opportunities.
- Facilitates an interdisciplinary process with other members of the healthcare team.
- Documents plan-of-care communications, rationale for plan-of-care changes, and collaborative discussions to improve patient care.

STANDARD 12. ETHICS

The radiology registered nurse integrates ethical provisions in all areas of practice.

Measurement Criteria:

The radiology registered nurse:

- Uses *Code of Ethics for Nurses with Interpretive Statements* (ANA, 2001) to guide practice.
- Delivers care in a manner that preserves and protects patient autonomy, dignity, and rights.
- Maintains patient confidentiality within legal and regulatory parameters.
- Serves as a patient advocate assisting patients in developing skills for self-advocacy.
- Maintains a therapeutic and professional patient–nurse relationship with appropriate professional role boundaries.
- Demonstrates a commitment to practicing self-care, managing stress, and connecting with self and others.
- Contributes to resolving ethical issues of patients, colleagues, or systems as evidenced in such activities as participating on ethics committees.
- Reports illegal, incompetent, or impaired practices.

Additional Measurement Criteria for the Advanced Practice Radiology Registered Nurse:

The advanced practice radiology registered nurse:

- Informs the patient of the risks, benefits, and outcomes of healthcare regimens.
- Participates in interdisciplinary teams that address ethical risks, benefits, and outcomes.

STANDARD 13. RESEARCH

The radiology registered nurse integrates research findings into practice.

Measurement Criteria:

The radiology registered nurse:

- Uses the best available evidence, including research findings, to guide practice decisions.
- Actively participates in research activities at various levels appropriate to the nurse's level of education and position. Such activities may include:
  - Identifying clinical problems specific to nursing research (patient care and nursing practice).
  - Participating in data collection (surveys, pilot projects, formal studies).
  - Participating in human subject protection activities, including informed consent.
  - Participating in a formal committee or program.
  - Sharing research activities and findings with peers and others.
  - Conducting research.
  - Critically analyzing and interpreting research for application to practice.
  - Using research findings in the development of policies, procedures, and standards of practice in patient care.
  - Incorporating research as a basis for learning.

Additional Measurement Criteria for the Advanced Practice Radiology Registered Nurse:

The advanced practice radiology registered nurse:

- Contributes to nursing knowledge by conducting or synthesizing research that discovers, examines, and evaluates knowledge, theories, criteria, and creative approaches to improve healthcare practice.
- Formally disseminates research findings through activities such as presentations, publications, consultation, and journal clubs.

STANDARD 14. RESOURCE UTILIZATION

The radiology registered nurse considers factors related to safety, effectiveness, cost, and impact on practice in the planning and delivery of nursing services.

Measurement Criteria:

The radiology registered nurse:

- Evaluates factors such as safety, effectiveness, availability, cost and benefits, efficiencies, and impact on practice, when choosing practice options that would result in the same expected outcome.
- Assists the patient and family in identifying and securing appropriate and available services to address health-related needs.
- Assigns or delegates tasks, based on the needs and condition of the patient, potential for harm, stability of the patient's condition, complexity of the task, and predictability of the outcome.
- Assists the patient and family in becoming informed consumers about the options, costs, risks, and benefits of treatment and care.

Additional Measurement Criteria for the Advanced Practice Radiology Registered Nurse:

The advanced practice radiology registered nurse:

- Uses organizational and community resources to formulate multidisciplinary or interdisciplinary plans of care.
- Develops innovative solutions for patient care problems that address effective resource utilization and maintenance of quality.
- Develops evaluation strategies to demonstrate cost effectiveness, cost benefit, and efficiency factors associated with nursing practice.

Standard 15. Leadership

The radiology registered nurse provides leadership in the professional practice setting and the profession.

Measurement Criteria:

The radiology registered nurse:

- Engages in teamwork as a team player and a team builder.
- Works to create and maintain healthy work environments in local, regional, national, or international communities.
- Displays the ability to define a clear vision, the associated goals, and a plan to implement and measure progress.
- Demonstrates a commitment to continuous, lifelong learning for self and others.
- Teaches others to succeed by mentoring and other strategies.
- Exhibits creativity and flexibility through times of change.
- Demonstrates energy, excitement, and a passion for quality work.
- Willingly accepts mistakes by self and others, thereby creating a culture in which risk-taking is not only safe, but also expected.
- Inspires loyalty through valuing of people as the most precious asset in an organization.
- Directs the coordination of care across settings and among caregivers, including oversight of licensed and unlicensed personnel in any assigned or delegated tasks.
- Serves in key roles in the work setting by participating on committees, councils, and administrative teams.
- Promotes advancement of the profession through participation in professional organizations.

Additional Measurement Criteria for the Advanced Practice Radiology Registered Nurse:

The advanced practice radiology registered nurse:

- Works to influence decision-making bodies to improve patient care.

- Provides direction to enhance the effectiveness of the healthcare team.
- Initiates and revises protocols or guidelines to reflect evidence-based practice, to reflect accepted changes in care management, or to address emerging problems.
- Promotes communication of information and advancement of the profession through writing, publishing, and presentations for professional or lay audiences.
- Designs innovations to effect change in practice and improve health outcomes.

References

American Nurses Association. (2001). *Code of ethics for nurses with interpretive statements*. Washington, DC: Nursesbooks.org.

American Nurses Association. (2003). *Nursing's social policy statement. Second edition*. Washington, DC: Nursesbooks.org.

American Nurses Association. (2004). *Nursing: Scope and standards of practice*. Washington, DC: Nursesbooks.org.

American Radiological Nurses Association (ARNA). (1998). *Standards of radiology nursing practice*. Oak Brook, IL: ARNA.

Morgan, L.K., & Nunnelee, J. (Eds.). (1999). *Core curriculum for radiological nursing*. Oak Brook, IL: ARNA.

INDEX

Q

R